The Top 10 Fat Loss Myths

J. Steele

Copyright © 2019
All Rights Reserved

BOOK TITLE

CONTENTS

Top 10 Fat Loss Myths i

    MYTH 1: SPOT REDUCTION WORKS 1

    MYTH 2: DRINKING COLD BEVERAGES REDUCES FAT 1

    MYTH 3: ELIMINATING FOOD GROUPS WILL CAUSE FAT LOSS 2

    MYTH 4: LOW CALORIE DIETS ARE THE ONLY WAY TO LOSE WEIGHT 2

    MYTH 5: YOU MUST WORK OUT AT SPECIFIC TIMES 3

    MYTH 6: YOU MUST WORK OUT FOR XX MINUTES BEFORE IT BEGINS TO WORK 4

    MYTH 7: EAT FAT BURNING FOODS TO LOSE WEIGHT 4

    MYTH 8: HIGH PROTEIN/LOW CARB DIETS ARE BEST 4

    MYTH 9: EAT LESS AND BURN MORE 5

    MYTH 10: ELIMINATE ALL FAT FROM YOUR DIET 5

AUTHOR NAME

BOOK TITLE

Top 10 Fat Loss Myths

Sticking to a diet is never easy, and with the abundance of weight loss myths circulating the weight loss community, it's often difficult to distinguish between effective weight loss techniques and strategies and misleading programs and tactics that are not only ineffective but often dangerous.

In this book, we'll cover the top 10 fat loss myths that have misled and confused dieters for years, so you can focus on realistic goals and surefire strategies of losing weight.

How many of these have you bought into?

MYTH 1: SPOT REDUCTION WORKS

It is widely believed that if you focus your exercise and weight training on specific areas of your body that you will be able to reduce the amount of fat in that specific area or region.

In reality, there is no such thing as spot reduction, and instead as you begin to work out and exercise you will start to lose weight evenly throughout your entire body.

Just the same, another common myth is that a high number of repetitions will burn more fat when in truth, fewer repetitions with a heavier weight will actually cause you to burn more fat in a shorter amount of time than a higher number of reps with a lighter weight.

MYTH 2: DRINKING COLD BEVERAGES REDUCES FAT

This is a very common myth that actually is believable if you consider the reasoning behind it.

The myth goes on to indicate that because your body needs to heat up the water, it automatically begins to burn calories whenever you drink cold water. This calorie burning frenzy continues until your body has adjusted the water temperature to be that of your regular body's warmth.

While drinking water (at any temperature) is an important part of any weight loss system, don't count on losing weight just from drinking alone.

Water helps flush out your system keeping you healthy and free of toxins, but you can not burn calories just by drinking it without a healthy diet.

MYTH 3: ELIMINATING FOOD GROUPS WILL CAUSE FAT LOSS

This myth is a bit confusing, so let's set the record straight.

Eliminating (or at least minimizing) certain foods such as foods that are high in sugars) should be part of your transition into healthy eating. You always want to minimize the number of high fat (low energy) foods whenever possible.

However, eliminating complete food groups from your diet and focusing on eating only one kind of food are not only very difficult to stick with, but in order to maintain a healthy diet, you need a well rounded selection of wholesome foods from all of the food groups.

Tip: Follow a well balanced diet that consists of foods from all four food groups, followed by a 'fat burning' turbulence training program for maximum results without sacrificing ANY of the foods you love!

MYTH 4: LOW CALORIE DIETS ARE THE ONLY WAY TO LOSE WEIGHT

Nearly every diet out there focuses on lowering your calorie intake and increasing your overall level of activity, and rightly so. The problem comes when dieters believe that by dramatically reducing their calorie intake they will shed the weight and keep it off.

It's important to gradually reduce your calorie intake so that your body's natural system doesn't shift into 'starvation' mode, which triggers your system into believing that you need to store food for a possible period of famine (this has been part of our system since the beginning of man).

You also need to watch out for a disruption in your body's natural metabolic pace, as dramatic reductions in calories can slow it down making it harder to shed those pounds.

MYTH 5: YOU MUST WORK OUT AT SPECIFIC TIMES

I've seen this myth circulate the weight loss communities many times over the years and while the "best time of day" always seems to change, the basic idea remains the same:

You need to work out at specific times for maximum results.

In reality, you really don't have to work out early in the morning, late at night or anything in between as long as you are actually exercising.

Focus more on maintaining a consistent schedule of activity and less on when you actually get it done.

For busy moms to business owners, being able to set a specific schedule isn't always the easiest thing to achieve, so it's great news that the real facts are that regardless of when you actually exercise, your body will burn the same amount of calories for the same workout regardless of the time of day.

MYTH 6: YOU MUST WORK OUT FOR XX MINUTES BEFORE IT BEGINS TO WORK

I used to believe this myth myself. The idea behind it is that your body must "warm up" for a period of time before it shifts into "fat burning mode", and so anything before xx minutes simply doesn't count.

This is complete nonsense! While you should always work towards incorporating a warm up period (as well as a slow down process) during your workouts, you actually start burning fat from the moment you begin!

MYTH 7: EAT FAT BURNING FOODS TO LOSE WEIGHT

If you ever truly find a food group or item that will cause instant weight loss, please, let me know!

Realistically, there are no foods that instantly burn fat, however there are food types that can increase your metabolism (which will subsequently, help you lose weight).

MYTH 8: HIGH PROTEIN/LOW CARB DIETS ARE BEST

These diets are typically difficult to stick with because they are very limiting in what you are allowed to eat. Furthermore, the reality of the matter is that while you may lose weight quickly at first, your body will plateau and you will find it difficult to get past the "hump".

Instead, focus on following a healthy eating plan that encompasses foods from the four food groups, ensuring that you not only are given added flexibility in your meal options, but that you are receiving the minerals and vitamins that your body requires.

MYTH 9: EAT LESS AND BURN MORE

Did you know what there is such a thing as a "Sumo Diet"? It's thought that Sumo wrestlers eat just before retiring for the day, and rarely eat throughout the day itself as a way of packing on pounds.

The reason for this isn't because eating after 7pm actually causes major weight gain (the number of calories you have stored at the end of the day will still be transformed into fat regardless of when you ate), but instead, they do this because when you eat less your body ends up storing more fat, while decreasing your metabolism rate.

It's important to eat regularly throughout the day, preferably 6-8 times (three meals and healthy snacks every two hours will keep you satisfied and trigger your body to stay in constant fat burning mode).

MYTH 10: ELIMINATE ALL FAT FROM YOUR DIET

This myth is not only extremely difficult to do, but it actually can harm your system. We all need fat in our diets to survive and to feed our muscles and encourage growth.

While reducing your fat intake will help you lose weight, it would be very difficult, if not impossible, to reduce it altogether.

Note: All of the weight loss resources and programs featured within this report are safe and effective. However, it is advised that you consult your family doctor prior to starting any weight loss program or weight training.

BOOK TITLE

BOOK TITLE

www.ingramcontent.com/pod-product-compliance
Lightning Source LLC
LaVergne TN
LVHW021751060526
838200LV00052B/3582